ORGANIC
EATING
THE
SAI WAY

ORGANIC EATING
THE
SAI WAY
Using
Sai-Entific
Methods

INDRA MOHINDRA O.D.

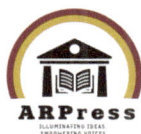

ARPress
ILLUMINATING IDEAS
EMPOWERING VOICES

ARPress

45 Dan Road Suite 5

Canton MA 02021

Hotline: 1(888) 821-0229

Fax: 1(508) 545-7580

Ordering Information:

Quantity sales. Special discounts are available on quantity purchases by corporations, associations, and others. For details, contact the publisher at the address above.

Printed in the United States of America.

ISBN-13:	Paperback	979-8-89356-434-1
	eBook	979-8-89356-433-4

Library of Congress Control Number: 2024904627

Table Of Contents

WHO IS SATHYA SAI BABA?

Who is Sai Baba? Many western readers, after reading my first edition of Eating Healthy the Sai Way, have asked me this question. I give them a simple answer: to me, He is my God and my Guru, my spiritual guide.

Sathya Sai Baba, when asked if He is God, responds: "Yes, I am God, and so are you. The only difference between you and Me is that while I am aware of this fact, you are not." Indeed, by giving this answer Swami is pointing to the fundamental truth of humanity's innate divine nature.

My ancestral heritage is deeply rooted in the ancient sacred scriptures of India, the Vedas. They teach very simple ways of living lives filled with truth, righteousness, peace, love, and non-violence. Through the Vedas, God gave mankind teachings on every aspect of life, from practical guidelines on health and diet (Ayur-Veda) to subtle spiritual wisdom. In the beginning, this wisdom was perceived directly by the Rishis. These highly evolved sages actually heard the words of the Vedas spoken by the Creator. For generations, the Rishis shared these teachings with their students and members of society. Gradually, with the passage of time, humanity began to ignore these teachings. At such dark times in human history, God (the supreme Divinity) manifests as an Avatar (Divine Incarnation) in human form, like Rama, Krishna, Buddha, and Jesus. The

Avatars incarnate with full divine power and knowledge to once again revitalize the essential values. Being an Avatar, the Creator Himself in human form, Sai Baba is also the author of the Vedas. So, His teachings about food are truly SAI: a Simple, Ancient, and Indian way of eating.

Just approaching my teens, I wanted my parents to go and search for the Avatar of our Kali Yuga (dark age)! Alas, I had to wait another thirty-four years before I found my Lord God, Sathya Sai Baba. It happened while I was watching a movie of His fiftieth birthday celebrations and heard Him say: "This year you have named My birthday the 'Golden Jubilee' of the Avatar!" Hearing the word "Avatar," I started sobbing uncontrollably! I also remember hearing His profound teaching: "My life is my message and My message is love.... The day when you resolve to practice My advice, to follow My directives, to translate My message into acts of service, and to engage in sadhana (spiritual practice)—that day is My birthday for you." Ever since that day my faith in His divinity settled permanently in my heart and not only did I read more of his teachings, but also I tried to understand and follow them implicitly.

Sai Baba was born on November 23, 1926, in Puttaparthi, Andhra Pradesh, India, a tiny village not then shown on any map whose population was not only less than five hundred but also relatively poor. He abandoned His schooling during eighth grade to start His Avataric mission. He discarded His physical body for His formless reality on April 24, 2011.

During the eighty-five years of His earthly advent, Sai Baba turned the small, invisible speck of His birthplace into a buzzing, booming city, a spiritual heart. Millions flocked to His hamlet from all over the globe, not only to taste the sweet nectar of His love, but also to get spiritually charged and transformed by His life of love and selfless service. They bore witness to His miraculous gifts: free educational institutions from KG (kindergarten) to PG (post-graduate) in various fields of study; free medical services offered through general, mobile, and super-specialty hospitals; and delivery of drinking water to quench the thirst of millions in southern India. As in the Vedas, Baba illumined every aspect of human life and spirituality, including health, as all facets are interconnected. In that spirit, I share with you my Sai food journey.

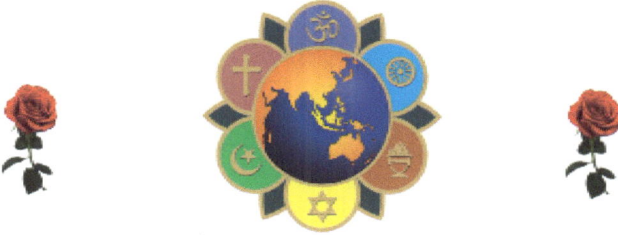

DEDICATION

I dedicate this book, recounting of my twenty years of food sojourn, accomplished at His command and under His Guidance, with Love and Devotion to Bhagavan Sri Sathya Sai Baba (Swami), in celebration of His 90th year of advent.

Swami always reminds me that I am a part of Him and not apart... He says, "I am always with you, never doubt that. Follow me. I am in you, with you, above you, beside you, and around you." To understand, experience and live these words of His is:

SAI - ENTIFIC EATING

DISCLAIMER

Based on Sathya Sai Baba's food guidelines, as experienced by me, this list is made to facilitate your choices for your daily meals. Your selections will be prompted by your health status in consultation with your medical providers.

ACKNOWLEDGEMENTS

I offer my gratitude to Bhagawan Sri Sathya Sai Baba for giving me full health after a nearly fatal attack of Asthma and granting me a gift of second life, on His 69th Birthday. He also guided me to follow His food journey and taught me that with a strong will power, patience, perseverance, and hard discipline, we can achieve most anything.

My thanks also go to all the Organic farmers and the organizations whose work helped raise my awareness of Organic and non-GMO foods and their health benefits not only for all humanity but also for all beings and for our planet's environment.

I sincerely thank my internist at Massachusetts General Hospital (MGH) Dr. Allan Goroll, M.D., who accepted me as his patient after my discharge from the Intensive Care Unit at MGH, in 1994. Under his excellent, compassionate and loving medical care, I was able to reduce the amount of medications and supplements, as my diet improved.

Indeed, I am very grateful to all my friends who very patiently listened to my food experiences at various stages of this journey and helped me with all my computer needs during my research and writing of this book.

Finally, to my dear mother who planted the vegetarian seed inside me from the day I was born and lovingly encouraged me about the follies of my change-over to a non-vegetarian diet. How proud she would be today, to see me in full health despite my advancing age, only by once again changing over to a wholesome, God-given, vegetarian way of life.

FOREWORD

Om Sai Ram

I am honored to write the foreword for this book that has presented a practical approach to the food we eat, based on Swami's teachings. The author's discipline towards food and her own experiences have inspired many devotees including myself.

I have known the author, Dr. Indra Mohindra, for over 30 years, during which period I have seen her go through several serious illnesses. Despite all those sufferings, she has gradually regained her health by making changes in her diet and habits as described in this book. She is a living example of the visible transformation that can be achieved by discipline, control of the tongue and implicit adherence to the words of our Swami. She did not wait for scientific evidence but took an early step following Swami's prescription faithfully, and this serves as a role model for the young and the old.

As a chemist, I have always admired the rhythmic biochemistry that Nature has created in the living beings. Our livers and kidneys are such tolerant organs that constantly work, handling all the food loads and the abuse we confront them with by our unhealthy eating habits. The agriculture and food industry; driven by greed has increasingly used a variety of pesticides, herbicides, hormones, antibiotics and genetic engineering that undoubtedly have subtle toxic effects on our organs.

The attractive processed "ready to eat" foods are geared toward marketing. The regulatory agencies cannot easily predict the long-term effects ofadditives, genetic modifications or chemical residues in foods until large randomized controlled studies, involving thousands of subjects, are conducted. But such studies are hard to design, very expensive to conduct and are very rarely done. Therefore, the frequently asked question on the scientific evidence remains unanswered.

It took several decades for the FDA to realize that partially hydrogenated oils used extensively in food products increase the bad cholesterol!

So, why feed toxins to ourselves and our children, while waiting for scientific evidence? Why not take our steps towards healthy eating by following Sai-entific guide-lines, as described by Dr. Indra Mohindra.This powerful small book has resulted from the author's own experience and extensive research of the literature.

This work of Dr. Mohindra is a 'wakeup call' for us to be constantly aware of keeping both the body and the mind pure for His service. It is not too late to change. Swami's words are nothing but the TRUTH.

Jai Sairam!

Shantha Sarangapani, PhD
President and Chief Chemist, ICET, Inc.
Massachusetts, USA

SWAMI'S QUOTES

The following of SWAMI'S quotes have been the guide posts during my two decade food sojourn, which I am sharing with you.

1. "HURRY, WORRY AND CURRY ARE THE CAUSES OF HEART PROBLEMS."

2. "Three Meals a day makes a man Rogi (Sick) - (Thamasic)
   Two Meals a day makes a man Bhogi (Enjoyer of food) - (Rajasic)
   One Meal a day makes a man Yogi (Healthy& blissful) - (Sathwic)"

3. "Put into practice what you hear."

4. "Practice what you preach."

"Old age is the fourth stage of life. By the time one reaches this stage of his journey he must have discovered that the joys available in this world are trivial and fleeting. He must be equipped with the higher knowledge of spiritual joy available through delving into the inner spring of bliss through his experiences; his heart must have softened and become full of compassion. He has to be engrossed in promoting the progress of all beings without distinction. He must be eager to share with others the

Indra Mohindra O.D.

knowledge he has accumulated and give them the benefit of his experiences."

Sathya Sai Speaks, Vol. 5 1984. Chapter 10

MY FOOD JOURNEY FROM SICKNESS TO HEALTH

I am very grateful to Sri Sathya Sai Baba for giving me a new life in November of 1994, when I was admitted to a hospital with my lungs nearly collapsed due to the medical diagnosis of chronic Asthma. I was in the ICU unit for four days and was released from the hospital on Swami's 69th birthday. A few weeks after that, He came to me in my dream and very emphatically told me, "No asthma, no asthma, no asthma! Stomach, Stomach, Stomach." The doctors could not diagnose any stomach ailment, and wanted me to continue with the standard treatment for asthma!

I knew that Swami's words could not be wrong, so while continuing with the excellent medical care, I contemplated as to what could be the cause of my stomach issues. Finally, I concluded that it was my, junky, vegetarian, diet (food from fast food chains, ready-made snacks and TV dinners, etc.) that was the cause of my stomach issues.

This revelation became firmer after further reading and digesting as much of Swami's literature on His health and food guidelines as my understanding and circumstances would allow. At first, I followed some of Swami's guidelines implicitly. I did not wait for scientific evidence for following these guidelines! Slowly I started to note a gradual improvement in my health, with less reliance on medicine.

However, some chronic symptoms still lingered on. So, my further research of His food literature led me to the most important teaching of eating only pure God-given food, not the man polluted and adulterated stuff which, under the shadow of so called scientific findings is poisoning our food. This is what Swami had to say:

"Due to an indiscriminate use of technology, the air, water, food, and everything is polluted and poisoned all over the world. Fortunately, the country of Bharat (India) is spared from this widespread pollution. We should not run after science and technology. Science without humanness is fraught with great danger to the very existence of humanity."

Convocation: Love is God, Live in Love, 22 November 2008, www. Sathyasai.

It is only recently I have started to implement this important teaching. The result is that I am enjoying fuller health benefits. With heartfelt gratitude to Swami, through this book I am sharing with you my experiences of gaining my better health, by following His guidelines. I call them SAI-ENTIFIC guidelines.

SAI-ENTIFIC FOOD GUIDELINES

•*Eat natural God given pure food*
• *Food gives health and illness.*
Listen to your body and stomach;
they will guide you to healthy eating.
• *Be a Lacto-Vegetarian.*
• *Eat no meat, fish or eggs. Drink no alcohol. Do not smoke, inhale, eat or drink any intoxicating food.*
• *Eat to live; do not live to eat.*
• *Eat in moderation.*
• *Eat only when hungry.*
• *Eat in a clean, calm, pleasant place, while seated and not while walking or talking.*
• *Eat in silence with your family and Without watching TV.*
• *Eat at least one meal of raw foods every day, perhaps for breakfast.*
• *Eat germinated, sprouted food.*
• *Do not eat processed, packaged-foods, with preservatives, artificial color, and chemical additives.*
• *Do not eat adulterated food such as white sugar, white rice, food sprayed with pesticides, herbicides or grown with chemical manures (non-organic) and genetically modified foods (GMO).*
• *Do not eat stale food.*

• *Do not take ice-cold drinks (sodas), some plastic bottled waters, and juices.*

• *Do not drink water with meals. Drink water half an hour before or half an hour after the meal. During the day drink eight - 8oz glasses of room temperature water, apart from that used in cooking, during the day.*

• *Do not eat yogurt or yogurt products for dinner or late in the evening or night.*

• *Do physical yoga. Vigorous exercise is not necessary if you eat optimum nutritional food.*

• *Raw food is healthy. Minimally cooked, slightly steamed or lightly stir-fried vegetables are healthier than over-cooked, over-boiled or fried.*

• *All vegetables and fruits should be well washed before peeling and eating.*

• *Grains and legumes (beans and lentils) should be soaked for at least half an hour or more, followed by thorough rinsing prior to cooking.*

• *Heaviest meal of the day should be lunch.*

• *Dinner should be a light meal, at least three hours before sleeping, followed by a half hour walk.*

• *Teens and adults should eat 2,000 nutrient dense calories and seniors (65 years and over) up to 1,500 nutrient dense calories per day. This intake of the calories can be adjusted according to the lifestyle of the individual.*

Environment, Timeliness, Moderation!!

SAI-ENTIFIC PROCEDURE FOR GOOD HEALTH

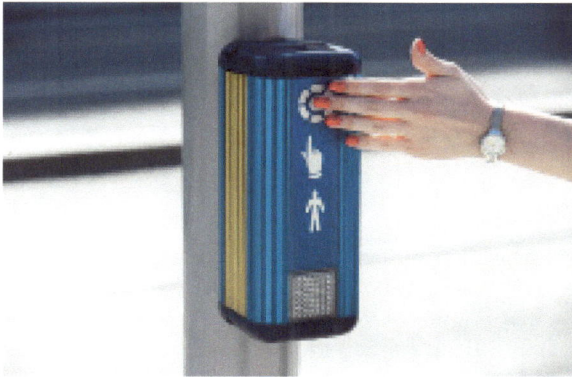

What I am sharing is not a fast and easy push-button method of healthy eating. I have learned to have strong will-power, patience, perseverance and discipline to follow this recipe of eating pure, wholesome God given food for good health.

"Discipline needs effort and will in the beginning, but becomes a habit with practice.... Discipline from outside is no discipline for the spiritual aspirant. Our thoughts and behavior at times must be self-monitored and self-enforced. It demands regular practice and belief in Swami's teachings. Swami's grace will always flow..."

Dr. Sara Pavan, Sydney, Australia, Sanathana Sarathi,

1994, Pg., 245

THREE IMPORTANT CONTROLS FOR COMPLETING ANY TASK

Swami has taught me that for accomplishing anything in this world, three things are essential:

1. Mastery over the senses.

2. Control over the mind.

3. Maintaining perfect bodily health.

Physically, the human body is a complex machine made up of six anatomical and physiological systems, the Skeletal, Muscular, Digestive, Respiratory, Cardiac Circulatory and Nervous Systems. The most vital of the six is the Digestive System, as it provides the needed energy for the smooth running of all others. God in the form of the fire (AGNI) resides in this system and helps with the digestion of the food we eat. However, spiritually human body is not one but three, Gross, Astral, and Causal. Residing in all the three bodies are the five enery sheaths (Koshas). These bodies are encased with the five energy sheaths. The five sheaths are; "foodstuff" (Annamaya Kosha), "energy" (Pranamaya Kosha), "mind-stuff" (Manomaya Kosha), "wisdom" (Vijnanamaya Kosha), and "bliss" (Anandamaya Kosha). The only visible sheath is the "food stuff" sheath, the physical body. All sheaths receive their energy from the quality and the quantity of the food we consume. The more

Sathwic (balanced) intake of our food, the closer we get to our ultimate goal of oneness with our Creator.

Food gives us body strength (health), which provides mental strength and results in improved spiritual strength, in Swami' words:

"Every activity of man is dependent on the energy he derives from the intake of food. The spiritual Sadhanas he ventures upon depend for their success on their quantity and quality of the food taken by the sadhaka (spiritual aspirant), even during the preliminary preparations recommended by Patanjali. The most external of the five sheaths which encloses the Atmic core, namely the Anamaya Kosha (physical sheath), has an impact on all the remaining four sheaths: the Praanamaya, the Manomaya, the Vijnaanmaya, and the Anandamaya (the vital, mental wisdom, bliss sheaths or coverings). The Manomaya is the sheath consisting of the material-flesh and bone- built by the food that is consumed by the individual."

21 September 1979, Sathya Sai Speaks, Vol, 14.

EMOTIONS AND FOOD ENERGY

The food we eat is subject to the infiltration of vibrations from the:

a) Source of food.

b) Environment such as watching TV, engaging in negative emotional conversations and unhygienic surroundings where food is cooked.

c) Emotions of the person who buys the food, the cook who prepares the food, the one who serves the food and the one who eats the food.

This control of the emotional energy of our food is critical for the proper assimilation to maintain good health of the body-mind complex.

Negative emotional effects can be neutralized when food is prepared in a spiritually-charged environment such as one in which one hears chanting of the Gayathri or singing of Bhajans (spiritual hymns). Also, prayer offering to God prior to eating our food helps to purify the vibrations the food.

Therefore, it is important to be constantly aware of the importance of the Sai-Entific guidelines.

"The mind is the key to health and happiness, and so food must be so chosen that it does not affect the mind adversely. Along with the sathwic food, the mind also is given a special diet like Dhyana (meditation), Japam, Namasmarnam (remembrance of the name of God), etc., to keep it sound and steady."

Sathya Sai Speaks Vol. VII, 1985, Chapter 16, Pg. 76.

FACTORS AFFECTING BODILY HEALTH

There are many internal and external factors which are important for maintaining good bodily health. These are nicely summarized by Dr. Raj Prakash8as follows:

1. FOOD AND WATER
2. EXERCISE, RECREATION AND SLEEP.
3. INNER AND OUTER ENVIRONMENT
4. THOUGHTS, EMOTIONS AND FEELINGS
5. INPUT FROM FIVE SENSES
6. GENETIC MAKEUP
7. PHYSICAL AND MENTAL POSTURE
8. EXPOSURE TO SUN
9. MEDICINE AND THERAPIES

However, the emphasis in this BOOK is on FOOD and WATER only.

"Food is essential for everyone in the world. Among the necessities of life food comes first. But man cannot be satisfied by food alone. A full stomach does not fully satisfy the mind. He cannot merely rest on a satisfied appetite. He has to move about and engage himself in work. While doing work, one has to ask himself: 'What am I doing? Why am I doing, and how am I doing?' When he delves into these questions and finds answers he can derive

meaning and joy from his work. In this way, he recognizes the purpose and value of what he is doing. Realizing what is good in his actions, he makes it a part of his life. He experiences the joy derived from his actions and shares that joy with others. This is the primary message of the Taittiiriya Upanishad. Starting with food, attaining bliss is the final goal of life."

Sathya Sai Speaks, Vol.24, 30 May 1991.

THE THREE TYPES OF FOOD

1. **SATHWIC** - Light and easily digested, producing calmness, equanimity and serenity. These foods are balanced and moderate, which are neither too hot nor too spicy, neither rajasic nor tamasic. They are easily digested and enable easy elimination. They help the mind to stay peaceful and tranquil and thereby are helpful for meditation and spiritual practices. Cow's milk, cream, cheese (unprocessed), butter, ghee, sweet fruits, vegetables, nuts, dried fruits, wholesome grains, raw (unrefined) sugars, ginger and raw honey are some of the often listed Sathwic foods.

2. **RAJASIC** - These foods produce too much energy and make one overactive, always on the go, and an enjoyment seeker. They also produce qualities like extreme anger, pride, conceit, egoism, arrogance etc. These foods are too hot, too spicy and too rich. Eggs, fish, meat, chilies, pickles, tamarind, sour things mustard, hot things, tea, coffee, cocoa, white sugar, carrots, turnips and spices are often listed as rajasic.

3. **TAMASIC** – These foods are the cause of inertia, lethargy, and sloth, also with the feelings of never enough sleep. These foods are insipid, too salty, too sour, too bitter and twice cooked foods. Beef, pork, wine, onions, garlic, rotten things, unclean things, alcohol, all intoxicants and drugs are often quoted in this category.

The ancient Indian food literature classifies food in the above cited categories; however, I have learned and experienced that the nature of the food consumed by us depends upon when, where, what type and how much we eat - as Swami teaches us that overfilling the stomach with Sathwic food can make it Tamasic.

"It is not enough if you eat good quality food alone. An excess of a good thing also becomes bad. Eating too much is rajasic, too little is tamasic. But eating the proper quantity is sathwic. So, one should learn to eat in moderation... Overeating causes diseases...one eats to live, one should not live to eat."

Sathya Sai's Amrita Vahini, pg. 11

THE PURE GOD-GIVEN FOOD IN KALIYUGA
(THE CURRENT ERA OF EXTREME DESIRES, DEPRAVITY, VIOLENCE, UNRIGHTEOUS ACTIONS)

Swami has often reminded us that Mother Nature is incredibly generous in the way she provides us her offering of a bounty of fruits and vegetables, rich in vitamins, minerals and nutrients, to nourish our bodies so we can enjoy a long, healthy life. Nothing concocted in a laboratory can ever replace the value of what is found in nature! So, it becomes clear that the pure God-given food cannot be the laboratory-produced food! In the current food-related literature two categories of food that come close to God given pure foods are:

1.   ORGANIC FOODS

2.   NON-GENETICALLY MODIFED (NON-GMO) FOODS. In some countries GMO foods are also known as Biotechnology or BT foods.

Every country has its own regulatory agencies that certify the organic and non-GMO foods, so it is recommended that individuals become aware of the symbols and authenticity of the products of the countries in which they reside.

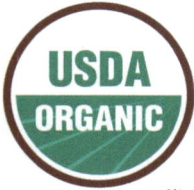

ORGANIC & NON-GMO FOODS

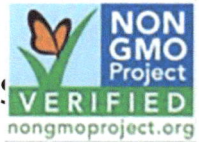

"Take fruits, which have nothing but vitamins, and vegetables, which can give you any amount of strength. What these give us today could be called artificial vitamins. In the old days, the common practice was to give plants manure in the natural state in the form of cow dung. The resulting vegetables might have been small, but they were rich in nutrients. Today, vegetables are oversized, and have lost their former flavor; what is the reason? Plants are now fed with artificial fertilizer, and they really do not have the innate strength which ought to be there. As a result, there is an increase in the cancer cases and heart complaints."

8th October 1983, Sathya Sai Newsletter, USA vol. 8-4

Organic foods are grown in soil with rotational crops and natural manure. They are grown or produced without the use of:

• Antibiotics
• Artificial growth hormones
• High fructose corn syrup
• Artificial dyes (made from coal tar and petrochemicals)
• Artificial sweeteners derived from chemicals
• Synthetically created chemical pesticide and fertilizers
• Genetically engineered proteins and ingredients
• Sewage sludge
• Irradiation

GENETICALLY MODIFIED ORGANISM (GMO) FOODS

"Whatever is given to the stomach, the stomach digests it and supplies the essence of it to all the organs. <u>This power of digestion given to stomach is</u>, in fact a God given thing. That is how one reveres and worships Him. In fact, God resides in a being as this digestive force, which is what governs and runs all the life processes in the body. To such a God as this, what is it that you should offer and give? This God should be given that which is His own creation, not which is made by man. So, whatever is available in the natural state, as given to you by God in His creation, if you want to give that to your stomach, everything will be all right." -- *Prashanti Nilayam, 10 August 1983. Transcribed by Estelle Tepper, edited by Diane Wells, June 1984*

GMO is an inter-species mixing (engineering) of genes from bacteria, viruses, fish, and animals which are inserted into the God-given genetic make-up of a plant, and sometimes they are chemically modified. These methods are different than previous techniques of Selective or Mutational breeding.

A few examples of foods that are now produced in the GMO form are cotton, tomatoes, zucchini, squash, sugar beets, corn, soya, alfalfa, canola oil, milk with rBGH (recombinant bovine hormone), rice, potatoes papaya and watermelons.

Tomatoes get fish genes inserted into their genetic makeup to increase their shelf life!

Corn gets genes from a bacterium known as Bacillus Thuringiensis or Bt into its DNA. Bt is a gram-positive, soil-dwelling bacterium, commonly used as a biological pesticide. Bt gene expresses a protein that kills insects, and transferring the genes to the corn allows it to produce its own pesticide!

Are seedless watermelons GMO? There are two types: one is a naturally occurring mutant, which occurs rarely; the second one whose genes are chemically altered by using a drug called Colchicine-a chromosome-altering chemical. This latter technique gives fast results to produce large quantities at the expense of poor quality.

Following Sai-Entific guidelines, what quantity and variety of the Organic and non-GMO food is available to us, to choose from?

DAILY SERVING REQUIREMENTS OF ORGANIC AND NON-GMO FOODS

Serving sizes for Lacto-vegetarians

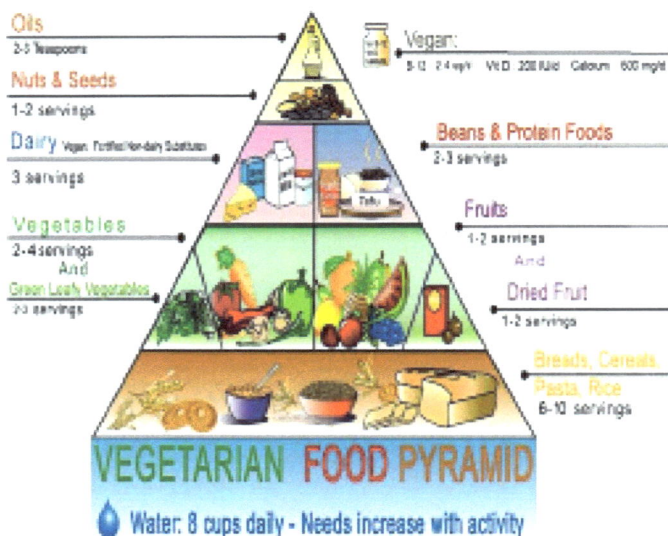

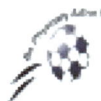

Oils
2-3 Teaspoons

Nuts & Seeds
1-2 servings

Dairy Vegan: Fortified Non-dairy Substitues
3 servings

Vegetables
2-4 servings
And
Green Leafy Vegetables
2-3 servings

Vegan:
B-12 2.4 ug/d Vit D 200 IU/d Calcium 600 mg/d

Beans & Protein Foods
2-3 servings

Fruits
1-2 servings
And
Dried Fruit
1-2 servings

Breads, Cereals
Pasta, Rice
6-10 servings

VEGETARIAN FOOD PYRAMID

Water: 8 cups daily - Needs increase with activity

© 2002 Department of Nutrition, Arizona State University
Art by Rick Richert

Sathya Sai Baba's serving sizes

What quantity of food is to be consumed to develop Sathwic qualities?

Swami gives us guidance to nourish this temple of God, our body.

Space in stomach is divided in 4 parts.

Youngsters, should fill 3 parts with food and one part with water.

Adult's, should fill 2 parts with food, one part with water & 1 part with air.

Filling all parts with food causes indigestion

USDA DAILY SERVING SIZE RECOMMENDATIONS

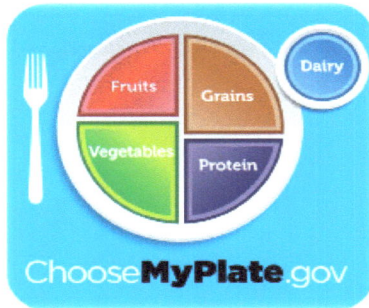

Vegetables: four servings
Fruits: three servings
Beans and Lentils: one serving
Dairy: two - three servings of milk or yogurt
Whole Grain: six - eleven servings
http://www.choosemyplate.gov

DAILY MENU SELECTIONS FROM NINE GROUPS OF FOODS

God has created a large variety of food for man to consume. It can become over-whelming to make good nutritional choices. I have put various foods in nine different categories from which to make our selection, according to our constitutional and metabolic needs. It is suggested that we select at least one or more items from each group, adhering to Sai-Entific guidelines, for our daily MENU, as per our daily caloric requirements. This will ensure a nearly perfect Sathwic diet.

1) Whole grains

2) Legumes - Beans / Lentils

3) Vegetables

4) Fruits

5) Nuts / Seeds

6) Spices, Salts, and Sugar

7) Oils / Butter

8) Dairy / Drinks / Water

9) Pickles

WHOLE GRAINS

- Pearl millet, Yellow millet (Bajra)
- Sorghum(Jawar), Red millet or Finger millet (Indian Ragi)
- Wheat, Spelt, Rye, Farro, Teff, Amaranth
- Bulgur Wheat (Cracked Wheat)
- Quinoa
- Brown Basmati, Brown Rice, Wild Rice, Black Rice
- White Rice (not good for Diabetics)
- Buckwheat
- Barley
- Oats

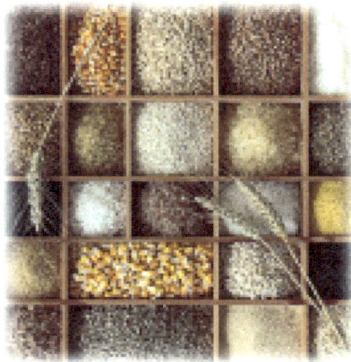

One should be aware of ethics in the use of grains. In the two countries where it is grown, global demand of quinoa is depriving the natives of their staple food. However, many other countries have started to grow quinoa. Also, some people may have allergies to some grains, like wheat - Gluten. These allergies may be due to excessive use of chemicals like Roundup (Herbicide), and many more. Also be aware of contraindications of some grains and foods with certain diseases and or medications. It is good to soak grains, lentils, and beans in water for at least half hour prior to cooking or even overnight. This process makes their digestion easier.

Instead of wasting the water used for soaking, you may use that water for your plants and thus providing them with nutrition. Water used for rinsing may be used this way as well.

LEGUMES – BEANS AND LENTILS

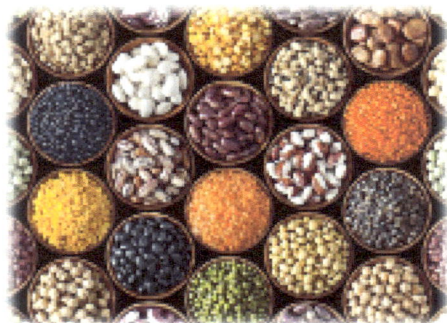

- Black Beans
- Black-Eyed Peas
- Fava Beans (Broad Beans)
- Chickpeas (Garbanzo), Black Channa
- Edamame Beans
- Kidney Beans
- Lima Beans
- Soy Beans
- Adzuki Beans
- Lentils – Moong (with and without skin), Masoor
- Lentils – French, Urad (with and without skin), Channa, Toor

This group of foods provides essential proteins for our diet. Black beans and French lentils are highest in their protein content. It is good to soak legumes for a couple of hours and drain the soaked water before cooking. It helps digestion.

GREEN LEAFY VEGETABLES - 'SUPER FOODS'

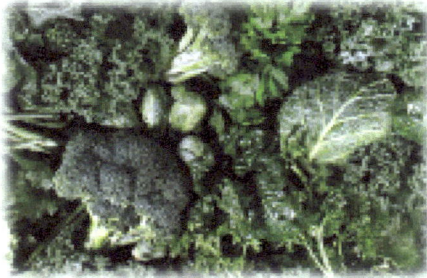

- Kale
- Mustard greens
- Collard greens
- Chard
- Spinach
- Daikon-Mooli greens
- Reddish greens
- Beet Root Greens
- Watercress
- Basil (Tulsi)
- Parsley
- Curry leaves
- Drumstick leaves
- Coriander leaves
- Mint leaves-Pudina
- Neem leaves
- Red & Green Cabbage
- Brussels Sprouts
- Methi-Fenugreek leaves

"THE DARKER THE GREENS, THE MORE NUTRITIOUS THEY ARE" - BABA

"Green leafy vegetables are the best of the lot. This is because under the human skin lies a very light secondary layer. It is this layer that protects the skin. Green leaves strengthen this layer, apart from having other benefits. It is very good for heart patients too because green vegetables are totally free of oils. Vegetables contribute to some extent to the cholesterol. What must you do when you have excess cholesterol? Cholesterol is essential to some extent. The limit prescribed is about 10%. But if it crosses 20% or 30% your nerves and arteries will harden like rusted pipes. This consequently thickens the blood making the heart pump less and less blood. The heart pumps the blood and sends it to the lungs which purify the blood and distribute it to the entire body. When the heart pumps less, more and more cholesterol accumulates there, which is dangerous for the heart."

http://www.saibaba.ws/teachings/foodforhealthy.htm

COLORED VEGETABLES

- Artichokes
- Turnips
- Parsnips
- Mushrooms
- Potatoes
- Tomatoes (without seeds)
- Kohlrabi, Okra
- Asparagus
- Onions (yellow, white, red)
- Garlic
- Ginger
- Arci (Taro Roots)

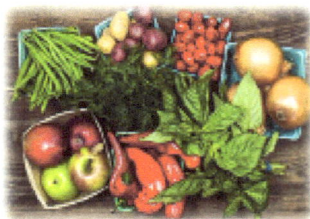

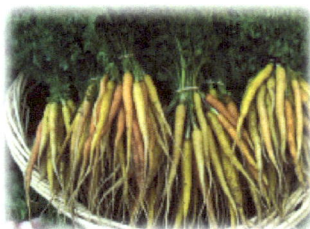

"In your hostel, there is of course no mutton and fish! But, onions are used extensively. This is because they do not get spoilt. Onion also has its advantages. It improves your digestion power."

"What must you do when you have excess cholesterol?...Take a white onion daily"

"Garlic pills can also be taken daily; a daily intake of one pill after lunch will get rid of the cholesterol problem. Green leafy vegetables and drumsticks are very healthy for the body. Drumsticks are good for the brain. Do not

take too much of potatoes. Potatoes contain 80 % starch that will only make you slightly fat, but also give you very little in terms of health. Tomatoes are also good. The seeds of the tomatoes may be removed and a curry made of the tomato. This is because the seeds of the tomato do not get digested easily. They remain in the digestive canal and gradually become stones, when they combine with glucose. These stones go down to the stomach and remain a mass, giving frequent trouble."

http://www.saba.ws/teachings/foodforhealthy.htm

SALAD GREENS AND SPROUTS

- Arugula
- Belgian Endive
- Lettuce
- Dandelion Greens
- Romaine Lettuce
- Baby Spinach
- Watercress
- Coriander Leaves
- Moong Bean and Other Lentil sprouts
- Wheat sprouts
- Soy Bean Sprouts
- Wheat Grass
- Chickpea (Garbanzo), Alfalfa sprouts

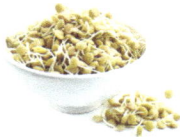

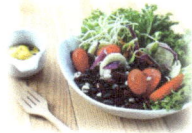

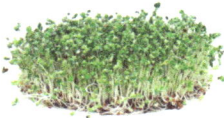

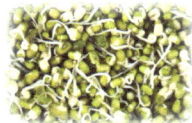

"Uncooked food, nuts and fruits, germinating pulses are the best. Use these at least at one meal, say, for the dinner at night. This will ensure long life. And, long life is

to be striven for in order that the years may be utilized for serving one's fellow-beings. Coconut kernel, coconut water , sprouting pulses, uncooked or half cooked vegetables, and greens are for good health."

Sathya Sai Speaks VOL X1 Pg. 149-151.

FRUITS

- Apple, Apricot
- Banana
- Berries - Black, Blue, Red
- Cantaloupe
- Cherries
- Cherimoya (Custard Apple)
- Citrus Oranges
  Tangerines
  Grapefruit
  Nectarine
- Coconut
- Date
- Fig
- Grapes - Green, Red, Purple
- Guava
- Kiwi
- Mango
- Papaya
- Peach
- Pear
- Plum
- Passion
- Pineapple
- Pomegranate

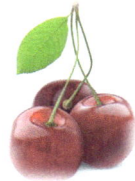

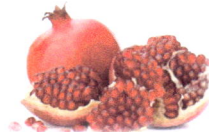

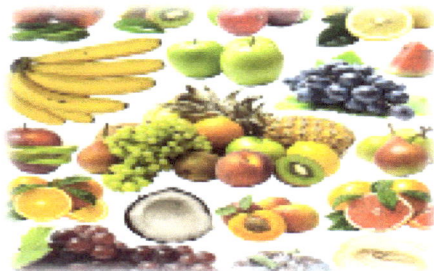

Eat fruit before a meal or on an empty stomach. Avoid cooking ripe fruit; cook only unripe fruit.

Watermelon is an excellent nutritional fruit, even diabetics can eat it. The seedless variety is a chemically altered mutant-GMO!

"Fruits with black seeds are very nutritional, except Cherimoya (Sitaphal) which has too much sugar."- Baba

"The coconut offered to God is a good sathwic (pure) food, having a good percentage of protein besides fat, starch and minerals."

21 September 1979, Sathya Sai Speaks, Vol 14.

DRIED FRUITS

- Apple
- Mango
- Cranberry
- Raisin
- Blackcurrant
- Fig
- Blueberry
- Prune
- Date
- Black Currants

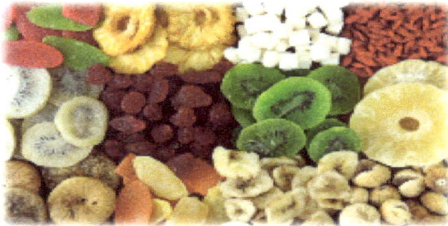

Before fruits are dried, they are often treated to preserve their color and prevent bacterial growth. The treatments may consist of natural substances, such as lemon juice and vitamin C, or they may consist of sulfur or sulfites. If you have asthma or you're allergic to sulfites, be aware of this and choose accordingly.

NUTS & SEEDS

- Hazel Nut
- Macadamia
- Walnut
- Pine Nut
- Pecan
- Almond
- Brazil Nut
- Cashew
- Water Chestnuts
- Pumpkin seed
- Sesame seed
- Sunflower seed
- Flax seed
- Chia seed
- Dill seed
- Fennel seed

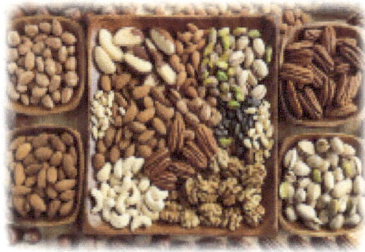

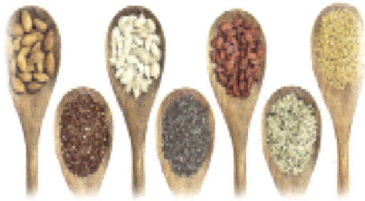

"... Fruits, and nuts, so forth; we understand to be Sathwic food. Food which is juicy, food that is oily, food that is tasty, delicious brings happiness on the physical plane. In this type of food there is something that has a subtle aspect to it, which sustains and really strengthens us. As far as possible this food should be associated with oil, but not with fat. We eat in limited quantities, to the

Indra Mohindra O.D.

extent that we can relish it... Food taken thus is truly Sathwic food."

25 July, 1983, Sathya Sai Newsletter, USA Vol 8-1.

DAIRY EQUIVALENTS AND WATER

- Whole milk (dilute with 50% water to reduce fat)
- Yogurt (made with diluted plain whole milk)
- Cottage Cheese, Paneer (made from whole milk)
- Soy milk (soy drink)
- Almond milk
- Rice milk (rice drink)
- Coconut milk
- Soy yogurt
- Cottage Cheese, Paneer (made from whole milk)
- Fermented Tofu (temphr)
- Sprouted Tofu
- Soy cheese
- Goat's milk
- Kefir (fermented cow's or goat's milk)
- Goat's milk cheese,
- Soy yogurt
- Eight glasses of water, boiled and cooled, at room temperature daily.

One should beware of aspartame (Nutra-Sweet or Equal), an artificial sweetener; it has been found to be carcinogenic and has been linked to many other diseases, besides cancer. It is commonly found in milk and some carbonated drinks, at sub-threshold levels, so legally it is not required to be listed on the label with other ingredients. Therefore, one might consider getting organic whole milk, from grass fed cows, who have not received any bovine growth hormones or antibiotics. Swami advises us to dilute this milk with 50% water which makes it easier for digestion. It is also recommended that we boil even the pasteurized milk before consumption, our ancestors always did that. He also advises us to avoid yogurt and yogurt products at night. Many processed foods are loaded with sugar; avoid them. Some fermented foods like idli, dosa, temphe, and some pickles are important sources of Vitamin K and B12; they should be a part of our diet.

"The older generation in this land used to take some quantity of rice soaked in curds as the first meal in the morning; it is a good Sathwic food; or they drank ragi gruel (finger millet porridge), which is very nutritious. Drink large quantities of water, boiled and cooled, not during meals, but some time before and after the meal."

Sathya Sai Speaks, VOL VII chap. 22 Pg 112.

SPICES

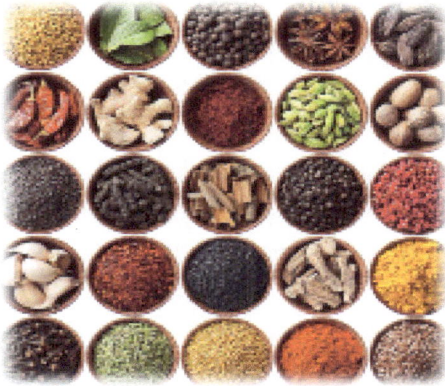

Cumin (jeera, jeerakam, geelakara)
Carom seed (ajwain, omam, ajumoda, vamu)
Coriander (dhania, kothamalli, dhaniyalu)
Caraway (jeera, sopu ginjalu, karinjirakam)
Fenugreek seed(methi dana, ventayam vital, menthulu)
Cloves (loung, lavangalu, kirampu)
Cinnamon (dalchini, ilavanka pattai, dalchina chekka)
Nutmeg (jayaphal, jatikkay, jajikaya)
Mustard seed (sarsokebija, katuku, avalu)
Black pepper (kali mirach, karrupu mimilaku, nalla miriyalu)
Saffron (kesar, kunkumappu, kunkuma puvvu)
Tamarind (imali puli, cintapandu)

Amchoor or Amchur (dried green mango or pomegranate seed powder)
Fennel seed (soumfa bija, perunchirakam vitai, sopu si)
Cayenne pepper (lal mirach, civappu milakay, karapu podi)

Spices are a valuable part of a healthy diet. The spices, give flavor to the food, can assist in its digestion, and often act as a preventive medicine. Swami says that humans often impair these functions by popping them while cooking in hot oil. Spices should be eaten in their raw form by grinding them into fine powder to sprinkle over the cooked food or to mix with hot or warm drinks. Fenugreek seeds soaked overnight in water and chewed first thing in the morning are beneficial for the eyes. Turmeric can be eaten in a variety of ways and provides antibacterial and anti –viral benefits. Many of the medicinal values and recipes for a variety of spices can be found in the attached link.

https://www.washingtonpost.com/lifestyle/wellness/spices-and-their-health-benefits/2014/01/07/4f074f26f2d11e3-aecc-85cb037b7236_story.html

SWEETENERS AND SALT

- Raw Cane Sugar
- Raw Honey
- Maple Syrup
- Indian Jaggery
- Coconut Palm Sugar
- Organic Vanilla Sugar
- Black Strap Molasses
- Stevia
- Sweet Brown Rice (Syrup)
- Sea Salt
- Mineral Salt
- Rock Salt (Kala Namak)
- Standard table salt

It is important to avoid artificial sweeteners and excessive salt. Both are detrimental for the health of the body. They are always found in processed foods. It is advisable to read the ingredient labels to detect their presence.

"Food having too much salt or pepper is Rajasic (passion-arousing) and should be avoided; so also, too much fat and starch, which are tamasic (promoting dullness and inactivity) in their effects on the body, should be avoided".

21 September 1979, Sathya Sai Speaks, Vol 14.

Indra Mohindra O.D.

"To this day, no one has come up with a solution for the problem of cancer. The cause of all this cancer is something worth knowing. Now, some might say that cancer is a direct result of smoking cigarettes. Others might say that air pollution is the cause. These factors might be contributing in a small way, but they are not the primary cause of cancer. The main cause of cancer is the white sugar. The reason for this is that, in the refining of sugar, a lot of chemicals are added. One of these processing chemicals is bone char, which, when you eat the sugar, [bone spicules] may get lodged in any part of the body and create problems...."

8 October 1983, Sathya Sai Newsletter USA, Vol 8-4

OILS

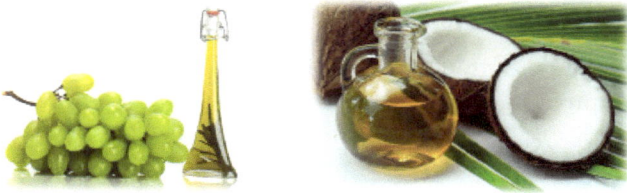

For Deep Frying: Avocado oil, Peanut oil, Rice Bran oil, Safflower oil, Sesame oil (light), Sunflower oil, Sweet Almond oil, Coconut oil, Grape Seed oil, Ghee(Purified Butter)

• **For Baking**: Coconut, Palm, Butter, Sunflower and Safflower.

• **For Frying**: Mustard, Peanut, Palm, Sesame (light), Ghee, Coconut (unrefined), organic Safflower, Sunflower, Corn & Grape-Seed oil, Avocado oil.

• **For Sauté-ing**: Avocado, Coconut, Grape Seed, Extra Virgin Olive Oil*, Sesame, High Oleic Safflower, Sunflower, Butter & Ghee-in moderation.

• * Extra Virgin Olive oil may have other oils like corn or canola oils mixed into it. These are added oils; therefore, one should avoid such impure olive oil. Buy olive oil in dak green glass ottles or packaging that shields it frm light.: avoid plastic containers. Exposure to light, heat, or oxygen can cause rancidity.

OILS

- Use Expeller Pressed or Cold Pressed oils and avoid oils processed with chemical solvents.

- Buy only Organic and non-GMO oils Canola oil is being sold as organic; however, it is always GMO. There is no canola plant seed. The seed is from a weed called Rapeseed, which is very poisonous in its natural wild state; even birds and animals will not eat it. The seed is genetically modified to get the oil. So growing it organically does not make it non-GMO.

- Avoid saturated from unsaturated fats. Unsaturated fats remain liquid in room temperatures. The saturated fat found in avocado and coconut is healthy when eaten in moderation.

- Avoid fried foods. However, if you choose to fry, always use fresh oil, because frying changes the oil to an unhealthy form. Be aware of allergies to some oils.

"As far as possible, the sathwic food should be associated with oil, but not with fat. We should eat in limited quantities, to the extent that we can relish it."

Sathya Sai News Letter, USA, VOL 28-3 (May-June2004)

"Sweet, sour, salty, hot and bitter...such items should not be taken in. Nor should we take in food that is absolutely dry and devoid of oil"

25 July, 1983, Sathya Sai Newsletter USA, Vol 8-4

"Til (sesame) seeds, rice flour and jaggery are mixed, made into balls, cooked in steam and offered to Vinayaka...Til (sesame) seeds are good for the eyes. Steam cooked preparations without any oil are good for your digestive system. One who partakes of such food will be free from high blood pressure and high blood sugar and will always enjoy health and happiness. Food items which are cooked in hot oil are harmful for digestion. Such foods are the cause of various diseases. One can lead a long, happy and healthy life if one avoids oily and fried foods."

31 August 1992, Sathya Sai Speaks, Vol. 8-1

SUMMARY OF GUIDELINES

1. EAT ORGANIC AND NON-GMO, FOLLOWING SAI-ENTIFIC GUIDELINES

2. AVOID PROCESSED AND PACKAGED FOOD.

3. WHOLE FOODS ARE BETTER IN ALL 9 GROUPS.

4. EAT ONLY WHEN HUNGRY; NO TV WHILE EATING; LISTEN TO YOUR BODY AFTER EATING.

5. EAT HIGH QULITY FOOD IN MODERATION; ADJUST QUANTITY WITH RESPECT TO YOUR LIFESTYLE AND AGE. EAT WHILE SEATED WITH NO TALKING.

6. NO ALCOHOL, CANNED OR SOME PLASTIC BOTTLED DRINKS.

7. DRINK EIGHT GLASSES OF WATER DAILY. SEPARATE FROM MEALS.

8. EAT AND LIVE IN A CLEAN & HEALTHY ENVIRONMENT.

10. DO ALL THE ABOVE IN CONSULTATION WITH YOUR MEDICAL DOCTOR AND YOUR INNER MEDICAL DOCTOR- -YOUR CONSCIENCE.

"In the food we eat, that which has the gross form of existence takes the form of excreta. The subtle part in the food takes the form of blood, and that which is intermediate between the gross and the subtle takes the form of muscles. What is the subtlest of all takes the form of mind. In the same manner, the gross form of water that we drink is given out as urine, while the subtle aspect of it gets transformed into Prana or life force. If food takes the form of the mind, and water the form of life force, you see how important it is what we choose to take in. If you do not exercise caution and control your diet, you cannot exercise control in your Sadhana (spiritual practices)."

25 July 1983, Sathya Sai Newsletter, USA, VOL 8-1

MY DAILY MENU SINCE AGE 75

As our bodies grow and change, our energy from our good food intake should also change. Swami says that we should be eating less quantity of good food as we get older. In my previous book, Experiencing Sathya Sai Baba, I wrote about my daily menu from age sixty to seventy. Now I am writing about my daily menu as of age seventy five.

Since age 75, I have started the day with an eight ounce glass of water at room temperature. My breakfast is four to five different types of fruits (seasonal if possible), five to ten almond nuts germinated by overnight soaking, and a cup of herbal tea. Two or three times during the week, after my fruits, I take porridge of oats made with diluted whole milk and a small quantity of organic sugar.

I am eating only one cooked meal a day, for lunch. I choose my menu from the nine food groups and include salads and yogurt. I drink no water with my meal, waiting at least until at least a half hour after the meal.

I end the day with a few selected nuts and dried fruits, or a sprout salad, only if I am hungry. I try not to take any snacks in between, except plenty of water. This has given me full health verified by my attached annual medical health report.

"People can live longer and (lead) more healthy (lives) if they eat only the minimum. Common sense, of course, is still necessary to ensure that with advancing age our body meets its nutritional needs. Sathya Sai Speaks, Vol. VII. 1985, Chapter,22. *"The intake of food should be gradually reduced after crossing fifty years."*

21 January1994, Sathya Sai Speaks, Vol. 27.

MY CURRENT MEDICAL REPORT SUMMARY

For the last four years I have strictly followed the above menu as per Sai-Entific Guidelines.

Below is a summary of my important Health results at age 78:

Blood Tests:
Oct 30, 2014, Nov 4, 2014

Allan Goroll, MD
Internal Medicine Associates,
Massachusetts General Hospital
Boston, MA. USA

Heart Disease HDL (Good Cholesterol)
LDL (Bad Cholesterol)
TRIGLYCERIDES
ANEMIA (Hemoglobin)
LIVER
KIDNEY
BLOOD PRESSURE 110/63

All these test results were well within **NORMAL LIMITS.**
My physician's comments:

"Your health is like that of a 23-year-old. Well, you will probably live to be 100!"

My reply: "But according to our scriptures our departure date was fixed on the day of our birth. No one knows or can predict that date!"

TESTIMONIALS

1. ALLERGIES AND DIET

I am a strict vegetarian and have been doing yoga and breathing practice (Pranayama) for over twenty years. This helped me sustain good health, but for one problem which I contracted eight years ago. I moved to the USA ten years back. All of a sudden, within a few years of moving to the USA, I started suffering from pollen allergy, during the moths of May and June. Each year doctors kept prescribing me a stronger dose of antihistamine medication. I started using an Ayurvedic NETI pot (a technique that helps to flush the nose with saline water), which helped a bit, but still I had to go on medication for almost all two months. This was troubling me. Thanks to Dr. Indra Mohindra, for giving us talks on following Swami's food guidelines and the role of organic and non-GMO foods for our health, I started monitoring my food intake. With strict discipline, my family and I completely shifted to organic, non-GMO food. For the past year, I am happy to say that I have refrained from taking any allergy medication and I am able to live a healthier life. This

has given me and my family a tremendous confidence in leading a healthy life.

Dr. Ramanan Ramanathan, PhD, MBA, Sharon, MA resident, a physicist by education and currently a cyber-security professional.

2. HEALTHY DIET

Our family being vegetarians, were eating a lot of rice and unhealthy food from restaurants that are high in fat and filled with cheese. As time passed, we became unhealthy. We decided to start eating healthy food but did not know how and where to start. At that time, we attended Dr. Indra Mohindra's talk on Swami's food guidelines. She mentioned the importance of organic food for health. The talks helped us to understand the benefits of eating healthy and how we should discipline ourselves into eating that food. We started changing our lifestyle to adapt to healthy eating. During this course, we consulted her many times and she even gave us some recipes and sometimes shared her healthy food with us. We found her instructions and we see a difference. We are healthy and happy and we are spreading the word whenever we can about eating healthy the Sai Way... Thank you Indra aunty for guiding us to be healthier and better people. Srikanth KT, SSE Education Coordinator, Sri Sathya Sai Baba Center of Walpole, MA, USA

3. ARTHRITIS AND DIET

"Take one step toward Me, I will take one hundred toward you."

Many years ago, I had a bout with arthritis (brought on by another illness). By God's grace, I went into remission. Having learned that traditional medications used for arthritis have potentially dangerous side effects, I looked into alternative methods. Diet was both the main culprit and the main cure. Meanwhile, my good friend Dr. Mohindra had great success applying Swami's directives on food - she had nearly left this world due to asthma but was now doing great by applying His teachings on diet.

I had minimal success making changes on my own (lack of self-discipline -- Indra would gently chide me for my horrendous sweet tooth). Several months ago, the arthritis worsened, particularly in my left hand and knees. It was time to take Swami seriously. Simply being vegetarian and eating fresh, unprocessed food was not enough; Indra suggested going on to organic and non-GMO foods. These can be expensive, but I was able to find affordable organics in the most unlikely places. Although I have not followed 100%, I have seen great results in just a few months. Not only is my hand much better (less pain, more range of motion), but also, I have lost 7% body weight, which helps my knees. All this from following Swami's teachings on food guidelines most of the time! Imagine what could happen if I (and everyone else) followed 100%! With gratitude to Swami and to Indra for, compiling and sharing this wisdom.

Rebecca, J. Jani, Vice President, Sri Sathya Sai Baba Center of Scarborough, Maine, USA.

4. PROTEIN FOR VEGETARIAN DIET

We have been tremendously lucky to have Dr. Indra Mohindra, give us very important suggestions on healthy eating according to Swami's guidelines. There are several instances where her advice was extremely useful. For instance, I have been particularly interested in eating a balanced diet that focuses a bit more on protein to help with strength training. In her book and talks she gave on this subject, I heard her mention the use of wholesome grains like wild rice, millet, and quinoa instead of white rice. She also mentioned that Swami makes us aware of the fact that all wholesome foods, some grains, vegetable seeds and nuts have a great deal of protein for us. So I made my dietary change by using a mixture of organic wild rice, millets and quinoa instead of white rice. This single change has helped me increase my protein intake by 20% while simultaneously reducing other starchy foods. It also brought to mind how Swami always said he ate just millet balls instead of rice as

His main food grain. Dr. Mohindra has worked really hard to bring Swami's teachings to the forefront. With all that is available to us in our grocery stores, she takes the guesswork out of shopping! I am sure that everyone will benefit from reading this book and making small and sustainable changes.

Ajay Yekkirala, PhD, Boston Children's Hospital, Harvard Medical School, Boston, MA, USA

SANKRIT PRAYER BEFORE EATING

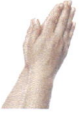

"FOOD IS GOD. IT CAME FROM GOD. MANY IMPURITIES IN FOOD WILL BE REMOVED BY OFFERING IT TO GOD. REMEMBER TO DO FOOD PRAYER PRIOR TO EATING YOUR FOOD".

http://www .sathyasai.org/devotion/prayers/brahmar.html

Prayer:

Brahmarpanam Brahma Havir Brahmagnau Brahmanaahutam Brahmaiva Tena Ghantavyam Brahmakarma Samadhina

The act of offering is God; the oblation is God. By God it is offered into the Fire of God, God is That which is to be attained by him who performs action pertaining to God.

Aham Vaishvanaro Bhutva Praninaam Dehamaashritaha Pranapana Samayuktah Pachaamyannam Chaturvidham

Becoming the life-fire in the bodies of living beings, mingling with the subtle breaths, I digest the four kinds of food.

Harir Daatha Harir Bhoktha
Harir Annam Prajaapatih
Harir Vipra Shareerastu
Bhoonkte Bhojayathe Harih

Oh Lord Hari, You are the food, You are the enjoyer of the food, You are the giver of the food. Therefore, I offer all that I consume at Thy Lotus Feet.

Swami's explanation of this prayer:

"We should partake food with a sathwic (pure, serene) mind. Our ancestors recommended the offering of food to God before partaking.

Food so partaken becomes Prasad (consecrated offering). Prayer cleanses the food of the three impurities caused by the absence of cleanliness of the vessel, cleanliness of the food stuff, and cleanliness in the process of cooking. It is necessary to get rid of these three impurities to purify the food, for pure food goes into the making of a pure mind.

It is not possible to ensure the purity of the cooking process because we do not know what thoughts rage in the mind of the man who prepares the food. Similarly, we cannot ensure the cleanliness of the food ingredients because we do not know whether it was acquired in a righteous way by the person who sold it to us.

Hence, it is essential on our part to offer food to God in the form of prayer so that these three impurities do not afflict our mind".

My experiences of listening to the body

1. With ingestion of tomatoes:

During the 1980's, I was residing and working in Boston, Massachussets, USA. My parents were living in London, England, UK. I would spend a couple of weeks of vacation during summer and Christmas with my parents. While staying with them I enjoyed my mother's Indian way of cooking my favorite recipes. Most Indian cooking is done with slices of tomato, onion, garlic and ginger. Tomatoes are also an important ingredient in the salads. I was really enjoying eating my mother's meals, reminiscent of my childhood days!

While my mother cooked, I spent my time knitting, which was my favorite pastime. There is no doubt I was enjoying knitting and enjoying my mother's cooking. However, after a few days of this eating routine, there was some pain in my finger joints. I blamed this annoying pain on my excessive knitting. But after coming back to my home in Boston, even with prolonged knitting, there was no pain. Reflecting upon this absence of pain, I could only relate it to my own non -Indian style of cooking which used very few tomatoes or none at all. Whenever I ate tomatoes the ache and pain in the joints would return. After becoming convinced that tomatoes were the cause of my aches and pains, I eliminated them from my diet. I avoided tomatoes from my diet for many years.

Recently, while reading Swami's discourses to His students, I noted His advice to them was to eat tomatoes without the seeds. Tomatoes, according to Him, are very nutritious; it is the seeds that are toxic. So now once again I am eating tomatoes without the seeds and there is no pain in my joints!

2. With ingestion of night shade family of food*

My father and his mother both had arthritis. Because of this family history, I have always taken an interest in investigating any preventive measure I could take to avoid this ailment of ageing. In addition to searching for Swami's food directives, I also researched scientific materials relating to the nutritional value of food. I was impressed by the writings of Dr. Joel Fuhrman, M.D. Many of his recommendations are vegetarian and are very similar to Swami's. He also provides food's nutritional values. While reviewing his material I discovered the high nutritional benefits of red, green and yellow peppers. As I wanted to increase my raw food intake, I started to add them in my salads. I knew that they belonged to the nightshade family and could cause arthritic symptoms. However, I ignored this as I was so impressed with their high nutritional value and taste, as well as the opportunity they offered me to increase my raw food variety. I started to eat them on a frequent and regular basis. Within a couple of weeks, I first noticed a slight irritation followed by a progressively swollen nodule on my right thumb. I consulted my internist who made the diagnosis of arthritis and referred me to a rheumatologist. The treatment included extraction of fluid from the nodule.

Upon hearing this I remembered Swami's quote that one's disease and health is related to the food we eat.

I immediately realized that the peppers in my new raw diet might be the cause of this current ailment! As my rheumatology appointment was a month ahead, I decided to delete the peppers from my food. As my appointment time was approaching the nodule was receding. A few days prior to my appointment it had completely disappeared. I kept my appointment with the rheumatologist, who questioned as to why I was even there! He said he had never heard of a story like mine and sent me home with a note that my thumb and I were very healthy.

*Nightshade Foods: potatoes, tomatoes, bell peppers, hot peppers, eggplants, huckleberries, pimentos, tomatillos, paprika, ground cayenne pepper and hot sauce and any other packaged food with any of these ingredients. It is very important to read labels and look for organic and NON-GMO foods.

3. With ingestion of wheat

Medically I have a history of asthma. Swami gave me the diagnosis of stomach ailment underlying the asthma. I continued with my excellent medical care but at the same time never had a doubt about Swami's diagnosis, as to me His words are the Truth! To me, He was the Doctor, and we were only His instruments. Already I had experienced two very successful previous surgeries, as per His advice. So after ruling out any possible medical causes of my stomach ailments, I reflected and meditated upon the causes for Swami's diagnosis. I got my answer fairly soon as I kept hearing in my head the word "food". Sure enough, even though I was a vegetarian, I understood that I was a "Junky Vegetarian". You see, at that time I was carrying a heavy load of part-time teaching and consulting with a few clinical practices spread out in the Metropolitan Boston area! This kind of lifestyle only gave me time for filling my stomach, to quench my thirst and appease my hunger I visited fast food places. I realized that the fast food was the cause of my stomach ailments. So I changed my habits by finding the time to cook my own food. Gradually, my physician and I started to see enough improvement in my breathing to reduce the dosage of my steroid treatment!

My healthy eating, over several years improved my general heath, but my lungs' air capacity showed a progressive deterioration. Normally, with increasing age, it is normal for the lungs air capacity to decline. However, in my case it came to a level lower than the expected norm for my age. During one visit, my medical doctor discussed the possibility of oxygen therapy, but decided to wait and confirm the reliability and stability of this reduced function, asking me to return for a follow-up visit in a couple of weeks.

Preceding this follow-up visit I came across an article on gluten sensitivity15. One of the symptoms could be breathing difficulty. I avoided wheat for the next few weeks and noted that my breathing was gradually improving. At the doctor's follow-up visit, my peak flow had doubled from its low value. The improvement I felt in my breathing was confirmed. Therefore, there was no need for oxygen therapy! I stuck with no wheat in my diet and replaced it with other grains. The result: my breathing has never again gone down below the age-expected norm.

One year after this episode I came across a scientific paper, from MIT's department of nutrition, questioning gluten in wheat as the cause of sensitivity or allergy and suggesting that a chemical in Roundup (glyphosate), which is sprayed over the growing wheat plants, could be the causative factor for the wheat sensitivity or allergies and not the gluten. The author explained that as some wheat plant's matured faster than others, at harvest the yield would certainly be increased if the younger greener plant's yield could also be captured. The use of Roundup did just that by killing the green leaves of the young plant so the kernel of this plant could also be extracted during the harvest, resulting in a higher total yield for the farmer. The agricultural industry paid no attention to the penetration of the toxic chemical into the wheat, the soil, the water as well as into the human cells of those who ate the Roundup sprayed wheat. I tested whether it was gluten or Roundup by eating chapatis (Indian tortillas) I made with organic wheat flour, that was not sprayed with Roundup but which of course still contained gluten, and I experienced no breathing problems!!!

4. With increased salt in my diet

I was in my mid-thirties and teaching at the University of Birmingham, in the state of Alabama, USA. I volunteered to be a patient for a student in a clinical laboratory session because of a shortage of patients for practicing his clinical procedures. After taking my blood pressure he informed me that it was high. I had it confirmed by one of my clinical colleagues. "Yes," said my colleague, "your blood pressure is high." I made an appointment with our cardiology department.

They also confirmed that it was high enough to consider medication. However, I hesitated to take medication so they asked me to return in a few weeks to see how reliable and persistent this high value was, before prescribing the medication.

At that time, I was a non-vegetarian. The red meat in southern states had salt as a preservative and at home more salt was added while cooking. Reflecting upon this, I sensed that perhaps meat and salt were the possible causes of my high blood pressure. So immediately I eliminated these two items from my diet. I continued with fish and chicken. I was not eating eggs because I was allergic to them. I was not aware of Swami or His teachings at that time. I just did it intuitively with my limited medical understanding of the nutritional needs. The result was that six weeks later, at my follow up visit with the cardiologist, my blood pressure had come down to a borderline level. Therefore, the cardiologist decided not to prescribe any medication for me.

The incident that made me a vegetarian occurred while watching a movie on television. I was not only horrified but disgusted to see a fish dying as they were trying to pull it out of the ocean waters. I felt the pain of the fish as it struggled for air when it was laid in a basket on the floor of the ship and then died. This affected my inner core and I vowed not to eat any animal beings for my food. I gave up eating fish, chicken and eggs and became a lacto-vegetarian! And this major dietary change took place before I had even heard of Swami. Reflecting on this now, I do understand that my becoming a vegetarian was, indeed, a call of my inner voice - - - that of my God, Bhagawan Sri Sathya Sai Baba.

5. Rash on my stomach

In the winter of the year 2013, I started to have a great deal of discomfort from dry skin. I had recently replaced my oil heating system with the gas. So, I installed a humidifier in my bed room. I got a slight relief. In addition to this I started oil messages, moisturizing creams and lotions. But all this failed to reduce my symptoms. By this time spring and summer had arrived, but the itchiness continued. Sometimes it was very severe.

I explored and ruled out any possible causative culprit in my environment like soaps and any other household cleaning agents or foods I might have unknowingly ingested. I was getting no clear answer.

At this point, a guest who was staying in my house alerted me to the fact that the water from my kitchen faucet had an odor and wanted to know if I could also smell it. I had not smelt this but I had questioned in my mind the yellowish discoloration of the water, which I had noticed sometimes but ignored. Now I realized that a year before I had installed a water filter that needed frequent replacements. I had forgotten to do so. This made me suspect that the odor my guest had noted and the yellowish color of the water could be due to the old filter. I started to think that perhaps some molds, fungus or bacteria from the old filter could be the cause of my itch and the rash on the skin of my stomach! Without wasting any more time, I had a plumber come and remove the filter. I convinced myself that because of the excellent quality of water in the Boston area, there was no need for the filter! I also made an appointment with my physician to consult about my symptoms. After a thorough medical testing to rule out any possible serious medical condition for my severely intense itchy rash, my internist finally referred me to a dermatologist, a skin specialist, who gave me a diagnosis of chronic eczema.

She explained that I needed a prescription of medicated moisturizing gel and a stronger steroid ointment to apply on the rash for brief periods of time during the flare-ups! She said I must learn to live with this condition.

I was very disappointed about this diagnosis and the recommended treatment. That night I prayed to Swami to guide me to find the cause of this problem. The more I contemplated and reflected about my situation, the more my inner voice prompted me to look into the foods I was eating. I searched for any difference in my eating habits prior to the itchy rash. Within a few days I discovered a couple of additions and omissions from my daily menu. According to my annual medical examinations over the past few years my health improved considerably, with a minimum of medications (inhalers for my lungs). I was taking these medications only when needed. As my health improved significantly, I started to ease up on my daily intake of dairy, flax seeds and aloe vera gel. Could the lack of these foods containing the anti-inflammatory nutrients be the cause of the inflammation in my body producing my symptoms? In addition, I had picked up some dark chocolate covered almonds from a store claiming all items for sale in their store were non-GMO and organic (as understood by me at that time). I had started to eat a few of these chocolates after my lunch as a desert. I have always had a weakness for chocolates. I read the ingredient label and found a few items that could have been non-organic or loaded with additives. After discovering this, I immediately threw away the remaining chocolates. Within two days of taking this action I noticed a reduction in the severity of the itch. A couple of days later I started eating the flaxseeds and drinking my daily dose of aloe Vera-gel. I also started taking my organic and non-GMO yogurt with my lunch. As soon as I started this new regimen in my daily menu, my itchy rash started to subside. After two weeks the rash and the itchiness almost disappeared! At this point I tried 100% organic non-GMO chocolate, this gave me no rash or itchiness!

Needless to say, I will continue to pay attention to my nutrient diet rather than take strong steroid medication! For me, eating not only an apple a day but also eating organic and non-GMO foods, keeps medication away.

CONCLUSION

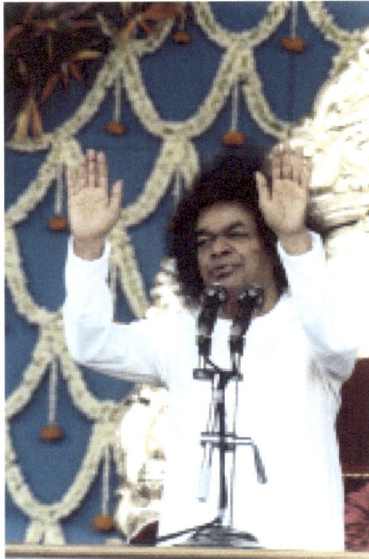

"Often when we lose hope and think this is the end, God smiles from above and says, 'Relax, Premaswarupalara, (Sweetheart), it's just a bend, not the end-- just keep taking that first step and I will take a hundred towards you."

JAI SAI RAM

REFERENCES

1. Compendium of the teachings of Sathya Sai Baba, Pg 134-141. Compiled by Charlene Leslie-Chaden, Third Edition 1998, ISBN 81-86822-19-4. printed at: D.K. fine Art Press (P) Ltd., Delhi India.

2. Sanathana Saraathi, September 2014, Supreme Bliss Comes from Absolute Wisdom, Bhagavan's Discourse: 1st September 1996, Eat only Pure and Sathwic Food, Pg 8- 10.

3. http://www.sairapture.com/chakra-bath.html BO Dr. Srikanth Sola.

4. http://www.amazon.com/dp/0984787208/ref=as_sl_pc_tf_lc?tag=sairap-20&camp=14573&creative=327641&linkCode=as1&creativeASIN=0984787208&adid=0Q9TT9QHJ5H2NB81KJE9&&ref-refURL=http%3A%2F%2Fwww.sairapture.com%2Fchakra-bath.html

5. http://0801.nccdn.net/1_5/15b/190/0f3/The Teachings of Sathya Sai Baba on Health - e-book.pdf

6. The Teachings of Sathya Sai Baba on Health, By Srikanth Sola, M.D. 1st edition 2000 2nd edition 2009

7. http://www.amazon.com/Eat-Live-Amazing-Nutrient-Rich-Sustained/dp/031612091X/ref=sr_1_1/179-4035469-9148657?s=books&ie=UTF8&qid=1422483673&sr=1-1&keywords=joel+fuhrman+eat+to+live

8. Swami on Health, Dr. Raj Prakash, Canton, Michigan, Sathya Sai Newsletter, USA, Fall1999, Vol. 24, Number 1. September, October, November issue.

9. http://gmosummit.org/former-pro-gmo-scientist/

10. http://gmosummit.org/former-pro-gmo-scientist/

11. http://www.biosciencetechnology.com/news/2015/09/people-who-eat-junk-food-have-smaller-hippocampi-australian-researchers-say?et_cid=4812756&et_rid=54752847&type=cta http://news.berkeley.edu/2015/09/15/bovine-leukemia-virus-breast-cancer/

12. EAT FOR HEALTH, Joel Fuhrman, M.D. Gift of Health Press, 2008.

13. MAN MANAGEMENT, A VALUES BASED MANAGEMENT PERSPECTIVE, BASED ON

14. The Discourses Of BHAGAVAN SRI SATHYA SAI BABA, Omkar Offset Printers, Bangalore,560092.

15. http://people.csail.mit.edu/seneff/ITX_2013_06_04_Seneff.pdf

16. http://thetruthaboutcancer.com/method-colorectal-cancer-screening/

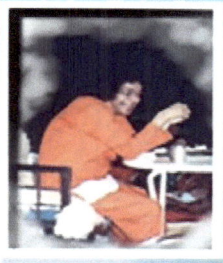

"People have read much, but how much have they applied their reading in life?"

Sathya Sai Speaks, Vol. IV, Pg. 164

In November 1994, a few days prior to Swami's 69 Birthday, the author suffered a near fatal illness (Asthma). Soon after this, in a dream visit Swami informed her that her illness was not due to Asthma but her stomach. In absence of any medical diagnosis confirming a stomach ailment, she pondered over her food habits.

Her conviction and faith in Swami's words, led her to not only read more of his food guidelines but to follow them implicitly. Over a span of twenty years of following Swami's Way of eating, she gradually noticed an improvement of her health and is finally enjoying full health, despite her advancing age.

In this booklet, she is sharing, with one and all, a simple and easy way to follow the Sai-Entific food guidelines by selecting from wholesome (organic and Non-GMO), pure God given food groups for our daily menu selection. The author has accomplished this only by following her beloved Bhagawan, Sri Sathya Sai Baba's valuable teachings.

SAMASTHA LOKA SUKHINO BHAVANTU.
(May all the beings in all the worlds be happy)